Title: No Fear of Sleep: Everything You Need to Know About Anesthesia

About The Author

Raúl is an anesthesiologist with over seven years of professional experience, dedicated to caring from behind the scenes. Originally from Spain, he has worked in both public and private hospitals, accompanying thousands of patients through one of the most delicate moments of their lives: the transition between consciousness and sleep, between uncertainty and trust.

His vocation was born from a deep desire to bring calm and safety just when everything seems to pause. With clinical precision and a quiet sensitivity, Raúl has come to understand that anesthesia is not just a technique; it is an act of care, a promise that everything will be alright.

This book is not only the result of his medical experience but also of his human perspective. It is a tribute to his profession, to the patients who have entrusted him with their lives, and to all those who choose to care without seeking the spotlight. Because in every anesthetic procedure, there is science, but there is also love, responsibility, and a quiet faith in the moment of awakening.

Introduction

It's the night before surgery. You've packed a small bag, signed your paperwork, and tried to distract yourself with TV. But as the clock ticks past midnight, one thought keeps returning: *"What if something goes wrong when I'm asleep?"*

This scene plays out for countless patients every day. Surprisingly, many people worry more about anesthesia than the surgery itself. The idea of surrendering consciousness, even for a short, safe period, feels deeply unsettling. Questions creep in: *Will I wake up? Will I feel pain? What if I lose control?*

These feelings are not only normal, they are nearly universal. Even confident, calm patients often whisper to their anesthesiologist: *"Please make sure I wake up."*

Here's the good news: anesthesia today is remarkably safe. Millions of patients receive it every year, and the overwhelming majority do so without complications. In fact, modern anesthesia is safer than many everyday activities, including driving to the hospital.

This book was written to take that worry you feel in the pit of your stomach and replace it with understanding. By the end of this chapter, you'll see anesthesia not as a frightening mystery, but as a powerful tool designed to keep you comfortable, safe, and pain-free.

Why Fear of Anesthesia Is So Common

Fear thrives where knowledge is missing. Anesthesia, by its nature, is invisible. You can't see it working, and you can't remember it happening. That mystery leaves plenty of room for anxiety.

Common Fears Patients Share

- *"What if I don't wake up?"*
    - *"What if I wake up too soon?"*

- *"What if I say something embarrassing while I'm asleep?"*
- *"What if the medicine affects me forever?"*

While these fears feel very real, medical evidence paints a far more reassuring picture. Out of a million patients, only a tiny handful face serious complications related to anesthesia, far fewer than most people imagine.

Think of anesthesia like dimming the lights in a room: everything goes quiet and calm so the surgeon can do their work. When it's time to wake up, the lights are gently turned back on. Behind the scenes, a highly trained anesthesiologist is carefully adjusting every detail to keep you safe.

Myths, Stories, and the Truth in Between

Because anesthesia is so mysterious, stories often take its place. A cousin who "woke up in the middle," a neighbor who "took forever to recover," or a dramatic TV episode that makes it all look terrifying.

Let's separate myth from fact:

- **Myth:** People sometimes don't wake up.
- **Fact:** With today's monitoring and medications, the risk is extraordinarily rare. Most patients wake up within minutes of surgery ending.
- **Myth:** You might feel everything but be unable to move.
- **Fact:** This is a common fear fueled by movies, but in reality, anesthesiologists use multiple layers of medicine and advanced monitoring to prevent awareness during surgery.
- **Myth:** Anesthesia damages your brain.
- **Fact:** For most patients, anesthesia has no long-term effects. Some older adults may feel groggy for a few days, but this is temporary.
- **Myth:** You'll say secrets under anesthesia.
- **Fact:** While sedation can make people a little chatty, the surgical team is focused entirely on your safety, not your words.

Knowing the facts not only dispels myths but also helps you see anesthesia as what it truly is: a life-saving gift of modern medicine.

What This Book Will Do for You

This guide is not written in medical jargon or complicated science. Instead, it's designed to:

- **Inform:** You'll learn what anesthesia is, how it works, and what to expect.
- **Empower:** You'll have tools, checklists, and questions to bring to your anesthesiologist.
- **Comfort:** Through patient stories, practical advice, and professional insight, you'll find reassurance.

Above all, this book aims to replace mystery with clarity. When you know what's happening, fear loses its power.

A Roadmap for the Journey Ahead

Here's how the book is organized to guide you step by step:

1. **The Basics of Anesthesia** – Clear, simple explanations of what anesthesia is and the types you may encounter.
2. **Preparing for Surgery** – How to manage nerves, what to tell your anesthesiologist, and what to expect.
3. **Inside the Operating Room** – A moment-by-moment look at what happens before, during, and after anesthesia.
4. **Recovery and Beyond** – Side effects, waking up, and safe healing.
5. **Special Situations** – Guidance for children, older adults, and patients with unique health needs.
6. **Your Questions Answered** – A section dedicated entirely to common fears and FAQs.

At the end of each chapter, you'll find practical checklists and questions to ask your care team.

Over the years, countless patients have leaned in with the same quiet request: *"Doctor, promise you'll wake me up."*

I always smile and answer, "That's exactly why I'm here."

And they always do, waking up safe, often surprised that the surgery they dreaded is already behind them.

Nurses, anesthesiologists, and surgeons all share this goal: not only to care for your body, but also to ease your mind.

Practical First Steps for You

If your surgery is coming up soon, here are a few ways to prepare right now:

- **Share your fears.** Tell your anesthesiologist exactly what's worrying you. Nothing is too small.
- **Write questions down.** Anxiety can make it easy to forget in the moment.
- **Bring support.** Having a family member or friend by your side can make the process less overwhelming.
- **Focus on the outcome.** Remember: anesthesia exists to keep you safe and pain-free.

Sample questions you might ask:

- What type of anesthesia will I have
- How will you monitor me while I'm asleep?
- What side effects should I expect afterward?
- How soon will I wake up?

Moving Forward with Confidence

Fear of anesthesia is normal, but it doesn't have to control you. With knowledge, preparation, and the reassurance of a skilled medical team, you can face surgery with far more confidence than fear.

This book will be your guide through every step, showing you that anesthesia isn't something to dread, but something to trust. You are not alone. You are cared for. And you are safe.

Part I: Understanding Anesthesia

Chapter 1: What Is Anesthesia?

Imagine this: you're sitting in a hospital gown, heart racing, waiting for surgery. A nurse tells you, "Don't worry, the anesthesiologist will be here soon." You nod, but inside your mind is buzzing with questions: *What exactly is anesthesia? Will I wake up? What if I feel pain?*

If this sounds like you, or someone you love, you're not alone. Fear of the "unknown" is one of the most common concerns before surgery.

The good news? You've already taken the first step toward calm by opening this book. In this chapter, we'll gently walk through what anesthesia really is, why it's used, where it came from, and why today's anesthesia is considered one of medicine's safest and most life-changing miracles.

So, What *Is* Anesthesia?

At its simplest, anesthesia is medicine that allows your body and mind to rest while doctors perform procedures that would otherwise be painful, frightening, or simply impossible.

Think of it like pressing "pause" on pain and awareness. Just as you dim the lights before going to sleep, anesthesia gently lowers your body's responses, sometimes just enough to numb a small area, sometimes enough to let your whole body sleep.

Doctors use different types depending on what you need:

- **Local anesthesia** – numbs a small spot, like when a dentist fixes a tooth.
- **Regional anesthesia** – numbs a larger area, such as during childbirth with an epidural.
- **General anesthesia** – allows you to sleep deeply while your entire body rests.

The goal is always the same: to keep you comfortable, pain-free, and safe during medical care.

A Quick Journey Through History

Believe it or not, people haven't always had this luxury. For most of history, surgery meant enduring unbearable pain. Ancient healers used alcohol, herbs, or even biting on a piece of wood to dull suffering.

That changed in **1846**, when the first successful public demonstration of anesthesia took place in Boston using ether gas. The news spread like wildfire; patients could now undergo surgery without agony. From that moment on, modern medicine took a giant leap forward.

Since then, anesthesia has become increasingly precise and safe. Today, anesthesiologists use advanced monitoring machines, finely tuned medicines, and years of specialized training to keep patients protected every step of the way.

The Miracle of Modern Anesthesia

Calling anesthesia a *miracle* isn't an exaggeration. Here's why:

- **Safety**: For every million patients who receive anesthesia today, only a handful experience serious complications. That's far safer than driving a car to the hospital.
- **Comfort**: Pain that once seemed unbearable is now preventable. Whether it's a C-section, a joint replacement, or delicate heart surgery, anesthesia makes it possible.
- **Precision**: Anesthesiologists can adjust your depth of sleep, level of pain relief, and even your body's response minute by minute.
- **Recovery**: Modern drugs wear off quickly, allowing patients to wake up smoothly, often within minutes after surgery.

What You Need to Know (and What's Just Nice to Know)

Need to Know:

- Anesthesia is designed to keep you pain-free and safe.
- There are different types depending on your procedure.
- Complications are extremely rare with today's technology and expertise.

Nice to Know:

- Anesthesia has a fascinating history stretching back to ancient times.
- Modern anesthesiologists spend years in training, mastering both medicine and patient safety.
- The science continues to advance, making procedures even gentler.

Questions You Might Ask Your Anesthesiologist

Bringing curiosity is a strength, not a weakness. Here are some questions you may find helpful:

- Which type of anesthesia will I need, and why?
- What side effects should I expect, if any?
- How will you keep me safe while I'm asleep (or numb)?
- When will I be able to wake up or move again?

Writing these down before your hospital visit can make you feel more prepared and confident.

Reassurance to Take With You

If you remember only one thing from this chapter, let it be this: anesthesia today is one of the safest aspects of modern medicine. Behind the science are compassionate doctors and nurses whose mission is to protect you, guide you, and bring you safely back to your loved ones.

By understanding what anesthesia is (and what it isn't), you're already transforming fear into knowledge. In the next chapters, we'll go deeper into specific types, safety measures, and how you can actively prepare for your anesthesia experience.

For now, take a breath. You're not alone, and you're in good hands.

Chapter 2: Types of Anesthesia Explained

When Maria (a patient) went in for knee surgery, she expected to be "knocked out cold."

To her surprise, we offered her options: "We can use general anesthesia so you'll sleep through everything, or we can do a spinal block that keeps you awake but completely numb from the waist down."

Maria blinked. *Wait, you mean I have choices?*

Many patients feel the same way. The word *anesthesia* often makes people picture only one thing: deep sleep. In reality, anesthesia comes in several forms, each designed for a specific purpose. Understanding the differences can take away much of the fear, because suddenly, it doesn't feel like an unknown anymore; it feels like a plan tailored to you.

This chapter will walk you through the four main types of anesthesia, when they're used, and what you can expect from each.

1. General Anesthesia – The Deep Sleep

Definition

General anesthesia is what most people imagine when they think of surgery: you're fully asleep, unaware, and pain-free while your body rests.

How it works (in simple terms):

Think of it as a carefully guided "power nap." Medicines are given through an IV or a breathing mask, and within moments, your brain drifts into a controlled sleep. Machines and monitors watch over your breathing, heart, and every vital sign while your anesthesiologist adjusts medications as needed.

When it's used:

- Major surgeries (heart, brain, abdominal)
- Operations that take a long time
- When complete stillness is important for safety

2. Regional Anesthesia – Numbing a Larger Area

Definition

Regional anesthesia blocks pain in a bigger section of the body while you stay awake (sometimes combined with sedation to help you relax).

Types include:

- **Spinal anesthesia** – medicine injected into the lower back, often used for C-sections or hip/knee surgeries.
- **Epidural anesthesia** – a continuous medicine drip through a small tube in the back, commonly used for labor and delivery.
- **Nerve blocks** – medicine placed near a specific nerve to numb, for example, just an arm or shoulder.

It's like flipping a circuit breaker that turns off electricity to one room of the house while the rest stays on.

When it's used:

- Childbirth (epidurals)
- Orthopedic surgeries (knee, shoulder, hand)
- Some abdominal or pelvic procedures

3. Local Anesthesia – The Small Spot Numb

Definition

Local anesthesia numbs only the exact spot being treated. You stay fully awake and aware.

Common examples:

- Dental fillings
- Stitches on a cut
- Minor skin surgeries

Think of it as using a tiny umbrella to block rain from just one patch of ground.

When it's used: Any quick, small procedure where full sleep isn't needed.

4. Sedation – "Twilight Sleep"

Definition

Sedation helps you relax and feel drowsy. It can range from light (you're awake but calm) to deep (you're sleepy and remember little or nothing). Sometimes it's called "twilight sleep."

How it feels:

Imagine dozing off in front of the TV—you're not fully asleep, but the world feels softer, calmer, less sharp.

When it's used:

- Endoscopies or colonoscopies
- Dental surgeries (like wisdom teeth removal)
- Short, less invasive procedures

Myth vs Fact

Myth: Anesthesia is "one size fits all."

Fact: Your anesthesiologist chooses the safest type for *you*, considering your health, surgery type, and comfort.

Myth: You might wake up during surgery.

Fact: With modern monitoring, this is *extremely* rare, less than 0.01% of cases.

Questions You Can Ask Your Anesthesiologist

- Which type of anesthesia will I receive and why?
    - Will I be fully asleep, partly awake, or just numb?
    - What are the most common side effects for my type?
    - Can I choose between options?
    - How will I feel after the procedure?

Quick Patient Prep Tips

- **Be honest about your health history** (allergies, medications, smoking, alcohol, etc.).

- **Ask about recovery time**—some anesthesia wears off faster than others.
- **Don't be afraid to express your fears**—your anesthesiologist is trained to answer them.

Reassurance to Take Home

Each type of anesthesia is like a tool in a carefully organized toolbox. Your doctors don't use the same tool for every job; they pick the one that best fits *your* body and *your* surgery.

Knowing the difference between general, regional, local, and sedation doesn't just inform you; it empowers you. You'll walk into the hospital not with fear of the unknown, but with confidence that your care is personalized, precise, and above all, safe.

In the next chapter, we'll dive deeper into **safety and monitoring during anesthesia**; the behind-the-scenes teamwork that keeps you protected every second.

Chapter 3: Meet the Anesthesia Team

When Olivia (another patient) came in for her gallbladder surgery, she expected to meet only the surgeon. But before she was wheeled into the operating room, I sat by her side, smiled, and introduced myself as the anesthesiologist.

I asked about her health, explained what medicines would use, and reassured him: *"My only job is to keep you safe and comfortable."*

It was the first time Olivia realized: surgery isn't just about the surgeon, it's about a whole team. And at the heart of that team is a group of professionals dedicated to one thing: making anesthesia safe.

If you've ever wondered, *"Who exactly is watching over me while I'm asleep?"*—this chapter is for you.

Who's Who in Anesthesia Care?

Anesthesia may seem invisible, but the people behind it are highly trained specialists. Let's meet them.

Anesthesiologists – The Medical Doctors of Anesthesia

- They are physicians (MD or DO) who specialize in anesthesia, pain management, and critical care.
- Training includes 4-6 years of medical school, 4-5 years of residency, and often additional fellowship training.
- Think of them as the "captains" of anesthesia care; they design the plan, make key decisions, and respond to emergencies.

If surgery were an airplane flight, the anesthesiologist is the pilot who ensures smooth takeoff, steady flight, and safe landing.

Nurse Anesthetists (CRNAs) – The Expert Nurses of Anesthesia

- CRNA stands for *Certified Registered Nurse Anesthetist*; They are advanced practice nurses who complete years of specialized anesthesia training.
- CRNAs provide anesthesia in many settings, such as hospitals, outpatient clinics, and even rural areas where doctors may not be present.
- In some parts of the world, they are the main anesthesia providers.

They're like highly skilled copilots: capable, experienced, and trusted to fly safely.

Anesthesia Assistants (AAs) – The Trained Partners

- AAs are professionals with a master's degree in anesthesia practice.
- They work under the supervision of anesthesiologists to monitor patients, adjust medicines, and assist during surgery.
- They are an important link in larger hospitals, where teamwork matters most.

They're like flight engineers, managing systems, double-checking equipment, and ensuring every detail runs smoothly.

How They Work Together

The anesthesia team doesn't work in isolation. They're part of the larger operating room family:

- **With surgeons**: They coordinate timing, discuss patient needs, and adjust anesthesia depending on surgical events.
- **With nurses**: They share vital information about your condition before, during, and after surgery.
- **With recovery staff**: They ensure you wake up safely, comfortably, and with good pain control.

Behind the scenes: While the surgeon focuses on the operation, your anesthesia team is solely focused on *you*—your breathing, your heart, your comfort, your safety.

Training and Expertise – Why You're in Skilled Hands

No matter their title, everyone on the anesthesia team is rigorously trained, licensed, and dedicated to patient safety. Here's a snapshot of the training pathway:

- **Anesthesiologists**: Medical school → residency → often subspecialty fellowships (like cardiac, pediatric, or pain medicine).
- **Nurse Anesthetists (CRNAs)**: Nursing school → ICU/critical care experience → graduate anesthesia program → national certification.
- **Anesthesia Assistants (AAs)**: Pre-medical background → master's program in anesthesia → certification under physician supervision.

What You Need to Know vs. Nice to Know

Need to Know:

- You will always have a trained anesthesia professional monitoring you, every second.
- Their entire role is to keep you safe and comfortable.
- They work as a team, not as individuals.

Nice to Know:

- There are different types of anesthesia providers, but all are highly trained.
- Anesthesiology is one of the most advanced and safest specialties in modern medicine.
- You can always ask to meet your anesthesia provider before surgery.

Questions You Might Ask Your Anesthesia Team

- Who will be with me during surgery?

- What type of anesthesia professional are you (doctor, nurse anesthetist, assistant)?
- What happens if something unexpected comes up?
- How will you manage my pain after surgery?

Quick Checklist for Patients

- Meet your anesthesia provider before surgery.
- Share your medical history honestly (allergies, medications, past anesthesia experiences).
- Write down your top questions ahead of time.
- Don't hesitate to express your fears—they've heard them all before.

Reassurance to Take With You

Behind every successful surgery is an unseen guardian; your anesthesia team. They may wear masks, but their mission is clear: protect you, comfort you, and bring you safely through the journey.

When you enter the operating room, you are never alone. A highly trained team is by your side, moment by moment, watching over you with both science and compassion.

And that's the heart of this book: turning fear into trust through knowledge.

In the next chapter, we'll explore what happens during anesthesia monitoring; the technology and watchful eyes that keep you safe every second of the way.

Part II: Before Anesthesia

Chapter 4: The Preoperative Assessment

When a patient walks into the hospital, an anesthesiologist is required to ask them several questions: "Do you smoke? Do you drink? Any allergies? Have you ever had surgery before?"

At first, you might wonder, *Why do they need to know all this?* But what you don't realize is that this conversation is one of the most important steps in keeping you safe.

This part of your surgical journey is called the **preoperative assessment**. It may feel like a lot of questions, tests, and checkups, but think of it as the medical equivalent of a pilot's pre-flight checklist.

Before the plane takes off, everything must be carefully reviewed to ensure a safe journey.

In this chapter, we'll explore what happens during this assessment, why honesty matters, and how it helps your anesthesia team tailor care just for you.

What Is the Preoperative Assessment?

The preoperative assessment is a thorough review of your health before surgery. Its main goals are:

- To identify any risks.
- To prepare your body for anesthesia.
- To create a personalized plan that keeps you safe and comfortable.

It's like a mechanic inspecting a car before a long road trip, checking the brakes, the tires, the fuel. The trip can't begin until everything is ready.

Step 1: Medical History and Physical Exam

Your anesthesiologist (or nurse anesthetist) will sit down with you and ask detailed questions. Don't be surprised if it feels like an interview; they're gathering information to protect you.

Topics often covered include:

- Past surgeries and any reactions to anesthesia.
- Allergies (to medications, foods, or even latex).
- Chronic conditions (like diabetes, asthma, heart disease).
- Medications, vitamins, or supplements you take.
- Lifestyle factors: smoking, alcohol, recreational drugs.

Afterward, you'll usually have a physical exam. The provider may:

- Listen to your heart and lungs.
- Check your blood pressure and oxygen levels.
- Look at your airway (to plan for safe breathing during anesthesia).

Step 2: Blood Tests, Imaging, and Risk Assessment

Depending on your health and the type of surgery, you may need tests such as:

- **Blood tests** – to check blood count, kidney and liver function, or blood sugar.
- **Imaging** – like a chest X-ray or heart scan if there are concerns about your lungs or heart.
- **Electrocardiogram (EKG/ECG)** – to look at your heart's rhythm.

These tests are like snapshots that give the anesthesia team more detail about how your body is functioning. Not everyone needs all of them; your doctor decides based on your health and surgery type.

The vast majority of patients pass these tests without issues. When something does show up, it usually just means the team adjusts the plan, not cancels the surgery.

Step 3: Why Honesty Matters

Here's the part where patients sometimes hesitate. You might feel uncomfortable admitting to smoking, drinking, or using recreational drugs. Or maybe you forget to mention herbal supplements because "they're natural."

But here's the truth: **your anesthesia team is not there to judge; they're there to protect you.**

- **Alcohol:** Regular use can change how your body responds to anesthesia.
- **Smoking:** Affects breathing and healing. Quitting even a few days before surgery can help.
- **Drugs or supplements:** Some can dangerously interact with anesthesia medicines or increase bleeding risk.

Key message: Being completely honest could be the difference between a smooth procedure and a dangerous complication.

What You Need to Know vs. Nice to Know

Need to Know:

- The preoperative assessment is routine, safe, and vital for your protection.
- Your anesthesiologist uses this information to create a personalized plan.
- Honesty about your habits and medications is critical; no detail is too small.

Nice to Know:

- Not every patient needs the same set of tests.
- Many issues discovered in the assessment don't cancel surgery; they just lead to adjustments.
- Even simple habits, like taking daily vitamins, can matter to your care team.

Practical Guidance for Patients

How to prepare for your preoperative assessment:

1. **Make a list of all medications and supplements** you take, including dosages.

2. **Be upfront about lifestyle habits** (smoking, alcohol, recreational drugs).
3. **Bring medical records** if you've had recent tests or specialist visits.
4. **Mention past anesthesia experiences**, good or bad.
5. **Write down questions** you want to ask (nerves can make you forget).

Questions you might ask your anesthesiologist:

- Will I need blood tests or imaging before surgery?
- How do my medical conditions affect anesthesia?
- Should I stop any medications or supplements before the operation?
- How long should I avoid eating or drinking before anesthesia?

Reassurance to Take Home

The preoperative assessment may feel like paperwork and questions, but in reality, it's your safety net. It's the step where your care team gets to know *you*;, not just your condition, but your body, habits, and history.

Remember: anesthesia isn't one-size-fits-all. Your honesty and cooperation allow the team to design a plan as unique as you are.

By the time you leave this appointment, you're not just a patient heading into surgery, you're a partner in your own care. And that partnership is one of the strongest shields against fear.

In the next chapter, we'll step into the operating room together and see how anesthesia is started and monitored, so you know exactly what happens once the journey begins.

Chapter 5: Common Concerns and Myths

The night before surgery, many patients find themselves lying awake, not because of the procedure itself, but because of the anesthesia.

Thoughts swirl: *"What if I don't wake up?"* ... *"What if I wake up too soon?"* ... *"Will I feel pain?"*

If you've ever had these fears, you're not alone. Nearly every patient has wondered the same things. These are deeply human worries, tied to our sense of control, trust, and the unknown.

The good news is this: modern anesthesia is incredibly safe, and the fears that feel overwhelming often have clear, reassuring answers.

In this chapter, we'll tackle the most common myths, separate fact from fiction, and give you the peace of mind that comes with understanding.

Myth #1: *"What if I don't wake up?"*

This is one of the scariest thoughts patients have. The idea of being aware while unable to move can feel overwhelming.

Fact: Intraoperative awareness is extremely rare, less than 0.1%.

Your anesthesia team continuously monitors your brain activity, heart, and breathing. If anything starts to change, adjustments are made instantly. Think of it like cruise control in a car: small corrections are happening all the time to keep the ride smooth and safe.

Myth #2: *"What if I wake up during surgery?"*

Hollywood movies love to scare us with this idea. In reality, anesthesia awareness (being awake during surgery) is *extremely rare.*

- **Fact:** It occurs in about 1 to 2 patients per 10,000, and most of those cases involve special high-risk surgeries where lighter anesthesia is used for safety (like major trauma or certain heart surgeries).
- Even then, patients usually do **not** feel pain.

Imagine falling into a deep sleep: sometimes you vaguely sense a noise but you don't really process it. That's the closest comparison to the rare cases of awareness.

Myth #3: *"Will I feel pain?"*

This is another very natural worry. Pain is something we all understand, and want to avoid.

Fact: Anesthesia's number one job is to keep you **pain-free during surgery**.

The anesthesiologist doesn't just put you to sleep; they also give pain-blocking medicines and adjust them as needed throughout the operation.

After surgery, they may also arrange for nerve blocks, epidurals, or strong pain relief so you wake up comfortably.

Think of anesthesia as a protective shield. While surgeons do their work, the anesthesia team makes sure you are not aware of pain and your body remains calm.

Myth #4: *"Anesthesia always makes you feel sick afterward."*

Many people believe nausea and vomiting are unavoidable after anesthesia.

Fact: These side effects can happen, but they are often mild, temporary, and easily treated with medication.

In fact, anesthesiologists often give preventive medicines before surgery if you're at higher risk. For most patients, recovery is smooth, and the feared sickness never comes.

Myth #5: *"Anesthesia causes permanent memory loss."*

Patients sometimes fear that anesthesia will permanently damage their brain.

Fact: Some temporary confusion or grogginess may occur, especially in older adults, but it usually clears within hours. There is no strong evidence that anesthesia causes permanent memory loss in healthy individuals.

It's like feeling foggy after a long flight—you may be a little disoriented at first, but your clarity returns once your body resets.

Myth #6: "*I can't have anesthesia because I'm allergic to medications.*"

People with allergies often worry that anesthesia is too dangerous for them.

Fact: True allergies to anesthesia drugs are rare. Anesthesiologists are trained to adjust your medications and choose safe alternatives.

It's similar to avoiding a food you can't eat—there are always other options available to keep you safe and comfortable.

Myth #7: "*Local anesthesia doesn't work well.*"

Some patients fear that local anesthesia won't block pain effectively.

Fact: Local anesthesia works very well for most people. If needed, it can be adjusted or combined with other forms of anesthesia.

Think of it as adjusting the volume on a radio. If it isn't quite right at first, your provider can simply "turn it up" or fine-tune it until you're completely comfortable.

Myth #8: "*Pregnant women can't receive anesthesia.*"

This myth can create unnecessary fear for expectant mothers.

Fact: Certain types of anesthesia are safe during pregnancy. For example, epidurals are routinely and safely used for cesarean sections, and general anesthesia can also be given when necessary.

Your anesthesia team carefully balances the health of both mother and baby, tailoring the safest plan for the situation.

Safety by the Numbers: Comfort in Context

Sometimes numbers bring comfort when explained clearly:

- **Not waking up:** less than 1 in 200,000
- **Awareness under anesthesia:** 1–2 in 10,000
- **Serious complication (in healthy patients):** less than 1 in 100,000

By comparison:

- The risk of dying in a car accident in the U.S. is about 1 in 8,000.
- Risk of being struck by lightning in a lifetime: 1 in 15,000.

In short: anesthesia is one of the safest parts of surgery.

How You Can Prepare Your Mind

Practical steps to manage your nerves:

1. **Write down your fears** and share them with your anesthesiologist. They've heard it all before and will gladly explain.
2. **Practice slow breathing** the night before—inhale for 4 seconds, exhale for 6. This signals calm to your body.
3. **Bring comfort**—a loved one's voice, a prayer, or even a favorite song in your head can help.
4. **Ask questions**—because knowledge reduces fear.

Sample questions you might ask:

- "How will you keep me asleep and safe?"
- "What will I feel when I wake up?"
- "What happens if I'm anxious right before surgery?"

Closing Reassurance: You Are in Good Hands

It's completely natural to feel anxious about anesthesia. But remember: anesthesia has advanced more in the past 30 years than almost any other medical field. With continuous monitoring, skilled teams, and proven medications, your chances of serious problems are extraordinarily small.

You are not alone in your worries, but you also don't face them alone. Your anesthesia team is with you from the first moment until you wake up safe and sound.

Knowledge replaces fear. And now, you hold the knowledge.

Chapter 6: Preparing Your Body and Mind

Imagine this: You've packed your bag for the hospital, laid out comfortable clothes, and tried to get some rest.

Yet your mind keeps racing: *What if I forget something? What if I eat by mistake? What if my nerves get the better of me?*

These thoughts are more common than you think. Nearly every patient feels a mix of anticipation and worry before anesthesia. The good news is that you can take concrete steps to prepare both your body and your mind.

These steps, like fasting, following medication instructions, and calming your nerves, aren't just "hospital rules." They are carefully designed to keep you safe and make your anesthesia smoother.

By the end of this chapter, you'll know exactly what to do the night before, the morning of, and even how to support your mind and spirit as you walk into the operating room.

Why Fasting Is More Than Skipping Breakfast

"Nothing to eat or drink after midnight"; you've probably heard this instruction before. But why does it matter?

When anesthesia puts you into a sleep-like state, your body's natural reflexes, like coughing or swallowing, take a break. If your stomach is full, food or liquid could travel upward and accidentally enter your lungs. Doctors call this *aspiration.* It's rare but serious. Fasting keeps your stomach empty and your lungs safe.

The basics of fasting before anesthesia:

- **Solid food:** Usually stop 6–8 hours before surgery.
- **Clear liquids (like water):** Allowed up to 2 hours before, unless told otherwise.

• **Chewing gum or candy:** Best avoided, as they can increase stomach acids.

Think of it this way: Just as you wouldn't drive a car with fuel spilling everywhere, your anesthesiologist can't safely guide you if your stomach isn't settled.

Medication Instructions: Which Pills to Take, Which to Pause

Not all medications play nicely with anesthesia. Some need to be stopped ahead of time, while others are crucial to continue.

• **Continue as usual (most of the time):** Blood pressure medicines, thyroid pills, heart medicines.

• **Pause or adjust:** Certain diabetes medications, blood thinners (like aspirin or warfarin), herbal supplements.

• **Special note on herbs & vitamins:** Natural doesn't always mean safe. Some, like ginseng or garlic, can thin your blood or affect anesthesia. Always tell your doctor what you take.

What you can do:

• Bring a complete list of all your medicines, including vitamins and herbal remedies.

• Ask: *"Should I take this pill the morning of surgery with a sip of water?"*

• Never guess. Clear instructions prevent last-minute confusion.

Calming the Mind: Practical Ways to Manage Anxiety

Fear before anesthesia isn't weakness; it's human. Even seasoned nurses admit to feeling nervous when they're patients themselves.

Here are proven ways to ease anxiety:

- **Breathing exercise:** Inhale slowly through your nose for 4 seconds, hold for 4, exhale through your mouth for 6. Repeat five times. It signals your brain to relax.
- **Mindfulness tip:** Imagine you're sitting on a beach, watching waves come and go. Each thought is a wave; let it pass without holding on.
- **Practical distraction:** Bring headphones and listen to calming music or an audiobook while waiting.
- **Talk it out:** Sometimes just telling the nurse, "I'm anxious," lightens the burden.

Special Situations: Tailoring Care to You

Not all patients are the same. Anesthesia is personalized—here's how it looks in certain groups:

Children

- Kids may be more afraid of being separated from parents than of surgery itself.
- Some hospitals let parents stay until the child is drowsy.
- Flavored masks, toys, or cartoons are often used to comfort them.

Elderly Patients

- Extra care is taken with heart, kidney, and memory health.
- Lower doses are often used to reduce grogginess afterward.
- Gentle reorientation ("You're in the hospital, the surgery went well") helps avoid confusion.

Pregnant Women

- Regional anesthesia (like an epidural) is commonly used for cesarean deliveries and is safe for both mother and baby.
- General anesthesia can also be given when necessary, with careful monitoring.
- Plans are tailored to protect both patient and newborn, with specialists always involved.

High-Risk Cases (e.g., heart disease, diabetes, obesity)

- More pre-op testing, like heart scans or blood sugar checks.
- The anesthesia team may consult with other specialists to fine-tune safety.
- Recovery plans are tailored to prevent complications.

Takeaway: Whether you're 5, 35 and pregnant, 50, or 85, your anesthetic plan is designed around you.

A Simple Pre-Surgery Checklist

Here's a handy list to keep in mind:

1. Stop eating at the instructed time.
2. Drink only clear liquids until cut-off.
3. Take only the medications your doctor approved.
4. Leave jewelry, nail polish, and makeup at home.
5. Practice a breathing or relaxation technique.
6. Bring your medication list and ID.
7. Tell the team if you're feeling especially nervous.

Closing Thoughts: You're Not Alone

Preparing your body and mind for anesthesia isn't about being perfect; it's about being informed. Every step, from fasting to calming your thoughts, is a way of partnering with your medical team for a safe, smooth experience.

Anesthesia today is one of the safest parts of modern medicine. With knowledge, preparation, and trust in your team, you can walk into surgery with confidence instead of fear.

Remember: Your questions are never a bother. Ask, share, and breathe; you are not alone in this journey.

Part III: The Anesthesia Experience

Chapter 7: The Day of Surgery

It's finally here; the day you've circled on your calendar. You arrive at the hospital or surgery center with a bag in your hand and a swirl of emotions in your chest.

Some patients describe feeling like they're waiting to board an airplane: a mix of nervous excitement, a few butterflies, and relief that the waiting is almost over.

You may wonder: *What exactly happens once I step inside? What will I see, feel, or hear?* These questions are completely normal.

This chapter is designed to walk you step by step through your surgical day; so instead of surprises, you'll have a roadmap.

What Happens When You Arrive at the Hospital

The journey begins long before you reach the operating room. Here's what most patients experience:

1. **Check-In at Reception**

You'll provide your name, ID, and paperwork. A nurse or receptionist will confirm details like when you last ate and what medications you've taken.

2. **Pre-Op Area (Preparation Room)**

You'll change into a hospital gown. A nurse will check your vital signs (blood pressure, pulse, oxygen level). This is also when an IV line, a thin, flexible tube placed into your vein, is usually started.

3. **Meeting the Team**

Your anesthesiologist or nurse anesthetist will visit you. This is your chance to ask last-minute questions like:

- "How will you keep me comfortable during surgery?"
- "What side effects should I expect afterward?"
- "How will you wake me up?"

Tip: Write down your questions ahead of time. Anxiety sometimes makes us forget what we wanted to ask.

Behind the Doors: Entering the Operating Room

Many patients imagine the operating room as intimidating, bright lights, masked faces, and machines everywhere. While it's true that the room is full of specialized equipment, every single item has one purpose: to keep you safe.

Here's what you'll notice:

- **The Lights:** Large overhead lamps make sure the surgical team sees clearly.
- **The Table:** Narrow but comfortable, often with arm boards so your arms rest securely.
- **The People:** A team working together; surgeons, anesthesiologists, nurses, and technicians; each with a defined role.

Think of it less as a "scary lab" and more as an orchestra. Everyone knows their instrument, and together, they create harmony to guide you safely through surgery.

Monitors, IVs, and Masks; What They Really Mean

Medical equipment can feel overwhelming at first. Let's break down the most common things you'll encounter:

The Monitors

- **Heart monitor (ECG):** Small sticky pads on your chest track your heartbeat.

• **Blood pressure cuff:** Inflates around your arm every few minutes like at the doctor's office.

• **Pulse oximeter:** A painless clip on your finger measures oxygen in your blood.

These monitors are your anesthesiologist's "dashboard," much like a car's speedometer and fuel gauge.

The IV (Intravenous Line)

Through the IV, your anesthesiologist can give you medicines, whether for relaxation, pain relief, or starting anesthesia. It's quick and efficient, and you may only feel a tiny pinch when it's placed.

The Mask

Sometimes you'll breathe oxygen or anesthetic gas through a soft mask placed gently over your nose and mouth. It's not tight or suffocating. One patient once described it as "like breathing in a cool breeze."

Myth vs. Fact:

• *Myth:* The mask will knock me out instantly.

• *Fact:* Often, anesthesia is started through your IV, and the mask is just for oxygen or gentle support.

Tips for a Calm Start

Here's how you can make the day go more smoothly for yourself:

• **Practice a calming breath** as you wait: in through your nose, out through your mouth.

• **Bring comfort items** (like glasses, dentures, or hearing aids) in a labeled case; you'll give them to the nurse before surgery and get them back afterward.

• **Tell your team about fears** whether it's needles, masks, or waking up. They hear these concerns every day and know how to help.

A Handy Checklist for the Day of Surgery

1. Arrive on time (hospitals run on precise schedules).
2. Bring only what you need: ID, insurance card, medication list.
3. Leave valuables at home.
4. Follow fasting and medication instructions exactly.
5. Share any new symptoms (like a cold or fever) with the team.
6. Remember: The monitors, IVs, and masks are there for your safety.

Closing Thoughts: You're in Caring Hands

Walking into the operating room may feel like stepping into another world, but it's a world built for your safety and healing. From the first monitor placed on your finger to the gentle oxygen you breathe through a mask, every step is carefully planned.

Anesthesia today is an extraordinarily safe process. Millions of people undergo it every year, and the vast majority do so smoothly and without complications.

As you lie back on the surgical table, remember: you are not just surrounded by machines, you are surrounded by people whose sole mission is to protect you, comfort you, and guide you safely through to recovery.

Chapter 8: Going Under

For many patients, the most anxiety-filled thought about surgery is this: "What will it feel like when I go to sleep?"

Some picture themselves drifting off gently, while others worry it will be sudden or unsettling. A few even ask, "What if I wake up too soon? What if I never wake up?"

These questions are completely natural. The transition into anesthesia is the moment that feels most mysterious because it's not something we experience in daily life. But here's the truth: for most people, it's easier and smoother than they ever imagined.

In this chapter, we'll walk through what actually happens when anesthesia begins, what patients typically remember (and what they don't), and the fascinating science of how the brain is gently guided into, and safely brought out of, this special state of controlled unconsciousness.

How Anesthesia Is Started

The process usually begins in one of two ways: through an **IV line** or through a **mask.**

- **IV Medications:** The most common method. The anesthesiologist gives medicine through your IV, and within 20–30 seconds, you feel drowsy, your eyelids grow heavy, and you drift off. Many describe it as feeling like a warm wave washing over them.
- **The Mask:** Sometimes used for children or adults who prefer not to start with an IV. You'll breathe oxygen, and sometimes a gentle anesthetic gas. The mask is soft, not tight, and the gas may smell slightly sweet. After a few breaths, the world feels far away.

Think of it this way: Going under anesthesia is like a dimmer switch being turned down on your consciousness. It doesn't flip off like a lightbulb, it fades smoothly until you're unaware.

What Patients Usually Remember (and Don't)

One of the strangest parts of anesthesia is how the brain stores, or doesn't store, memories during the process.

What patients often remember:

- The pre-op area, talking to nurses and doctors.
- The moment of getting the IV or feeling the mask.
- Sometimes a nurse asks you to take deep breaths.

What patients usually don't remember:

- The exact moment they "go under." Most people are mid-sentence when their memory stops.

- Anything from the surgery itself. The brain is safely shielded from forming memories.

- Waking up in the middle; this is an extremely rare event (less than 1 in 20,000 cases in modern anesthesia).

The Science of Losing and Regaining Consciousness

Your brain is like a city at night: full of lights, signals, and communication between neighborhoods. Anesthesia works by gently quieting those signals.

- **Falling Asleep Under Anesthesia:** Medicines slow down activity in the parts of the brain that control awareness and memory. Unlike natural sleep, you don't dream or shift positions. It's a carefully managed pause.
- **Staying Safe During Surgery:** Throughout, monitors track your heart, breathing, and oxygen. The anesthesiologist adjusts medicines as needed, like a pilot adjusting altitude during flight.

• **Waking Up:** When surgery ends, the medicines are reduced or stopped, and your brain "lights up" again. Most patients open their eyes within minutes and can answer simple questions.

Unlike fainting or being knocked out, anesthesia is a controlled, reversible process, one that doctors can fine-tune every second.

Myths vs. Facts About Going Under

• Myth: "I might wake up during surgery."

Fact: With modern monitoring and medicines, awareness is extraordinarily rare.

• Myth: "I won't wake up afterward."

Fact: Millions of anesthetics are safely given each year. Healthy adults have extremely low risks, and even higher-risk patients are carefully managed.

• Myth: "Anesthesia is like natural sleep."

Fact: It may look similar, but anesthesia is deeper and more controlled, with no dreaming or tossing and turning.

Practical Tips for a Calmer Experience

• **Trust the routine:** Remind yourself that your anesthesiologist has guided thousands of patients through this exact process.

• **Use breathing techniques:** Just before the IV or mask, take a few slow, deep breaths to calm your body.

• **Share your fears:** Whether it's "I'm afraid of needles" or "I don't like masks," your team can often adjust to make you more comfortable.

• **Focus on the next step—not the whole journey.** Tell yourself, "Right now, all I need to do is lie back and breathe."

Questions You Might Ask Your Anesthesiologist

• "How exactly will I go to sleep?"

- "Will I feel anything during surgery?"
- "How do you make sure I wake up safely?"
- "What will I remember afterward?"

Asking these questions doesn't annoy your doctor; it reassures you and helps them know what matters most to you.

A Short Checklist Before Going Under

1. Share your fears honestly with your anesthesia team.
2. Practice one relaxation technique (breathing, visualization).
3. Remind yourself that going to sleep usually feels smooth and easy.
4. Remember: your anesthesiologist's number-one job is to bring you back safely.

Trust in the Transition

The moment of "going under" may feel mysterious, but it's one of the most carefully studied and safest parts of modern medicine. For most people, it feels like closing your eyes for a brief moment and then opening them to find it's all done.

As you take that last deep breath before anesthesia, remember: you are in skilled, watchful hands. This is not a leap into the unknown; it's a guided passage, and your team is there to carry you safely through it.

Chapter 9: Behind the Scenes While You Sleep

Imagine this: You close your eyes in the operating room, and the next moment you remember is waking up in recovery. To you, it feels as if time disappeared.

But behind the scenes, an entire team, and especially your anesthesiologist, was wide awake, carefully guiding your body through every second.

Many patients worry, *"Once I'm asleep, what if something goes wrong and no one notices?"* This chapter is here to show you just how closely your body is monitored, how anesthesia doses are adjusted with precision, and how your safety and comfort remain the team's top priority.

Continuous Monitoring: The Safety Net That Never Sleeps

From the moment you go under until the moment you wake up, you are never left unobserved.

What's monitored:

- **Heart:** Sticky patches on your chest send signals to a screen, showing every beat.
- **Breathing:** A small tube or mask measures how much oxygen and carbon dioxide move in and out of your lungs.
- **Blood pressure:** A cuff inflates regularly to make sure your circulation is stable.
- **Oxygen levels:** A tiny clip on your finger, glowing red, checks how much oxygen is in your blood.

Think of it like flying on an airplane: while you relax in your seat, the pilot's eyes are glued to the dashboard. Your anesthesiologist does the same, constantly scanning your "dashboard of vital signs."

Adjusting Doses: Fine-Tuning Every Step

Anesthesia is not "one size fits all." It's a living process, adjusted second by second.

- If your blood pressure dips, medicines can be given to bring it back up.
- If your body shows signs of stress (like a faster heart rate), more anesthesia or pain relief can be added.
- If your body is stable, doses may be reduced to avoid unnecessary medicine.

Imagine adjusting the water temperature in your shower. Too hot, you turn it down. Too cold, you turn it up. Anesthesia is fine-tuned in much the same way to keep your body in the perfect balance.

Managing Pain and Vital Signs Together

Anesthesia isn't only about keeping you unconscious; it's about making sure your body is comfortable and protected.

What's happening while you sleep:

- Pain signals are blocked so your brain doesn't register discomfort.
- Muscles may be relaxed to allow the surgeon to work more safely.
- Fluids are given through your IV to keep your circulation steady.
- Medicines are adjusted to prevent nausea after surgery.

Myth vs. Fact:

- *Myth:* "I won't feel pain because I'm asleep."
- *Fact:* Sleep alone doesn't block pain, but anesthesia does, using carefully chosen medicines.

How You Can Prepare and Feel Reassured

Even though you won't be aware of these behind-the-scenes efforts, knowing about them can help you feel calmer. Here's what you can do:

- **Before surgery:** Ask your anesthesiologist, *"How will you monitor me while I'm asleep?"* Hearing it explained can be very reassuring.
- **During pre-op:** Share your health history honestly; conditions like asthma, diabetes, or heart disease guide how monitoring and medicines are tailored to you.
- **Trust the team:** Remind yourself that modern monitoring technology and trained experts work together like layers of safety nets.

A Patient's Quick Checklist

1. Ask what monitors will be used during your surgery.
2. Tell your team about any past anesthesia experiences (good or bad).
3. Share if you have sleep apnea or use a CPAP at home.
4. Remember: monitors are not there because something is wrong; they are there to keep everything right.

Safe in Skilled Hands

While you sleep, your anesthesiologist is wide awake—listening to every heartbeat, watching every breath, and guiding every moment. The machines are important, but it's the skilled human watching those screens that makes all the difference.

So when you let go and drift into anesthesia, remember: you are not "on your own." You are cared for, second by second, by a team whose sole mission is your safety.

Part IV: After Anesthesia

Chapter 10: Waking Up

Imagine this: You blink awake and notice soft lights overhead. A nurse is nearby, gently calling your name.

For a split second, you might wonder, *"Is it over already?"* That's often the first surprise; many patients say it feels like no time has passed at all.

For some, waking up from anesthesia can be confusing or even a little unsettling.

Will I feel pain? Will I remember where I am? These are natural questions.

In this chapter, we'll walk through what recovery feels like, what's completely normal, and how the medical team keeps you safe every step of the way.

What Recovery Feels Like

Waking from anesthesia is not like waking from a regular night's sleep. It's more like slowly surfacing from underwater. You may drift in and out before fully realizing you're in the recovery area. Here's what you might notice:

- **Grogginess**: Feeling sleepy or heavy-headed is the most common effect. Think of it as your body "rebooting."
- **Nausea**: Some people feel queasy, but medicines are available to ease this quickly.
- **Sore throat**: If a breathing tube was used, your throat may feel scratchy for a day or two.
- **Chilliness or shivering**: Your body temperature can dip slightly under anesthesia, but warm blankets and monitoring take care of this.
- **Mild pain or discomfort**: The surgical area may feel sore, but pain relief is usually started before you're even fully awake.

Most of these sensations fade within hours, sometimes minutes.

How the Team Keeps You Safe

Just because you're asleep doesn't mean your care stops; it actually shifts gears. When you wake up, you're in the **Post-Anesthesia Care Unit (PACU)**, sometimes called the recovery room.

Here's what happens behind the scenes:

- **Continuous monitoring**: Nurses track your breathing, oxygen, blood pressure, and heart rate.
- **Gentle wake-up process**: Your anesthesiologist carefully times the reduction of anesthesia so you don't wake up too suddenly.
- **Pain management**: Medications are given based on your needs, often started before you even ask.
- **Nausea control**: Anti-nausea medicine can be given if needed.
- **Family updates**: In many hospitals, once you're stable, your loved ones are informed or allowed to visit.

Practical Guidance for Patients

Here's how you can prepare for the recovery experience:

- **Before surgery, ask your anesthesiologist**:
    - "What can I expect when I wake up?"
    - "How do you manage nausea or pain after anesthesia?"
    - "When will I be able to see my family?"
- **Bring comfort items**: Lip balm, glasses, or a small personal item for after surgery can help you feel grounded.
- **Plan for grogginess**: You'll need someone to take you home, and you shouldn't drive or make big decisions for at least 24 hours.

Reassurance and Empowerment

Recovery from anesthesia is carefully managed and closely supervised. While you may feel groggy, scratchy-throated, or a little queasy, these are normal and temporary sensations. What's more important is that your surgical team is watching over you, making sure your first moments awake are safe and as comfortable as possible.

Remember, anesthesia is not just about putting you to sleep; it's also about waking you up gently and safely. With knowledge, preparation, and trust in your care team, you'll find that this stage, too, can be handled with confidence and calm.

Chapter 11: Pain Management After Surgery

Imagine this: you've just had surgery, the hardest part is over, and as you slowly open your eyes, the first thought that crosses your mind isn't about the procedure itself; it's about the pain. *"How bad will it be? Will I be able to handle it?"*

You're not alone in this. Almost every patient has some fear of pain after surgery. It's natural. Pain is the body's way of saying, *"I've been through something big."* But here's the reassuring truth: modern medicine has more tools than ever to help you recover with comfort and safety.

This chapter will walk you through those tools: medications, nerve blocks, even non-drug approaches, and show you how doctors carefully balance pain relief with your overall safety. Most importantly, you'll learn how to talk openly about pain so your care team can support you better.

What Do We Mean by "Pain Management"?

Think of pain management as having a toolbox. No single tool fixes every problem, but when you combine the right ones, the job gets done smoothly. Doctors don't just reach for one option; they often use a multimodal approach, which simply means using different methods together.

Here's what might be in your pain-relief toolbox:

- **Medications** – These can range from simple options like acetaminophen (Tylenol) to stronger pain relievers like opioids, carefully dosed and monitored.
- **Nerve Blocks** – Imagine turning off the "power supply" to pain signals in a specific area of your body. A nerve block does just that, numbing the region for hours or even days.

• **Non-Drug Approaches** – Ice packs, gentle movement, relaxation techniques, or even listening to calming music: all of these can reduce discomfort.

Each method plays its part, and together, they create a smoother, safer recovery.

The Balancing Act: Comfort and Safety

One of the biggest concerns patients have is: *"Will I be given too much medicine?"* or *"Will I become addicted?"*

Here's the fact: your care team's job is to balance comfort with safety.

• Too little pain control can slow down your recovery; you may not want to move, breathe deeply, or eat well.

• Too much medication, especially opioids, can bring side effects like nausea, sleepiness, or constipation.

That's why anesthesiologists and nurses keep a close eye on you, adjusting the plan as needed. You're never expected to "tough it out" in silence, but you also won't be given more than your body needs.

Talking About Pain: Why Your Voice Matters

Pain is personal. What feels like a "2 out of 10" for one person may feel like an "8" for another. That's why hospitals often use pain scales, asking you to rate your pain from 0 ("no pain") to 10 ("worst imaginable pain").

Don't worry about being "too dramatic" or "too stoic." Your honest answer helps your team fine-tune your care. *"We can only treat the pain we know about."*

Practical Tips: How You Can Take Charge

Here's how you can make your pain management plan work better:

• **Speak Up Early**: Don't wait until pain becomes severe; tell your nurse as soon as it starts rising.

- **Know Your Options**: Ask about alternatives; "Can I try a nerve block?" or "Would non-opioid medicines be enough for me?"
- **Be Honest**: If you're worried about side effects or addiction, say so. Your doctor will respect and address your concerns.
- **Try Non-Drug Helpers**: Bring headphones, calming music, or a relaxation app for your hospital stay. Small things make a big difference.

Questions you can ask your anesthesiologist:

- "What's your plan for my pain after surgery?"
- "Will I need opioids? If so, how long?"
- "Are there non-medication options that could work for me?"
- "What should I do if I feel over-sedated or too drowsy?"

The Takeaway: Comfort Without Fear

Pain after surgery is real, but suffering doesn't have to be. With today's multimodal strategies, doctors aim to keep you comfortable enough to heal, move, and rest, while keeping you safe from unnecessary risks.

Remember: pain management is a partnership. When you speak openly, your care team can guide you toward a recovery that's not just about getting better, but also about feeling better along the way.

So as you prepare for surgery, take this to heart: you are not alone, and you do not need to be afraid of pain. With knowledge, communication, and trust, comfort is well within reach.

Chapter 12: Possible Side Effects and Complications

Many patients, upon waking from anesthesia, whisper the same words: *"Is this normal?"* Whether it's nausea, shivering, or a scratchy throat, the first sensations can sometimes spark worry.

If you've ever wondered, *"What side effects should I expect? What's serious, and what's not?"*; you're asking the right questions. Feeling nervous is natural.

The good news is that most side effects after anesthesia are temporary, mild, and treatable. Serious complications are very rare, and your care team is trained to catch and treat them quickly.

This chapter will guide you through what you may feel after anesthesia, why it happens, and which warning signs to watch for once you go home. By the end, you'll know what's expected, what's unusual, and when to ask for help.

Common, Mild Side Effects: The "Normal Bumps" of Recovery

Nausea and Vomiting

- **Why it happens**: Anesthesia medicines can sometimes irritate the stomach, and surgery itself can trigger queasiness.
- **How it feels**: Think of it like motion sickness; it's uncomfortable but usually short-lived.
- **What helps**: Doctors often give anti-nausea medicine before or after surgery. Sipping clear fluids and starting with light foods afterward can also make a big difference.

Shivering and Feeling Cold

- **Why it happens**: The body cools slightly during surgery, and anesthesia affects how your brain regulates temperature.
- **How it feels**: Some patients wake up shaking or with teeth chattering, even under warm blankets.
- **What helps**: Nurses can use warm blankets, heated air devices, or medications to calm the shivers. Most patients stop shivering within 15–30 minutes.

Sore Throat or Hoarseness

- **Why it happens**: If a breathing tube was used during surgery, your throat may feel scratchy afterward.
- **How it feels**: Similar to a mild cold or after cheering loudly at a sports game.
- **What helps**: Lozenges, warm liquids, and gentle care usually relieve it in a day or two.

Rare but Serious Risks: Putting It Into Perspective

It's natural to worry about "what if something goes wrong." Here's the comforting perspective:

- Out of **a million patients**, only a handful face serious complications from anesthesia.
- Modern monitoring and safety standards have made anesthesia **safer today than ever in history**.

Still, it's important to know the possibilities:

- **Allergic Reactions**: Very rare, but doctors keep emergency medicines ready just in case.
- **Breathing or Heart Problems**: More likely in patients with existing heart or lung conditions, which is why pre-surgery evaluations are so detailed.

- **Awareness During Surgery**: Extremely rare, affecting about 1–2 people in every 1,000. If it happens, patients usually recall sounds or pressure but not pain.
- **Nerve or Dental Injury**: Rare complications linked to positioning or airway management.

Warning Signs After You Leave the Hospital

Most patients recover smoothly at home, but here are signs that should prompt a call to your doctor, or in urgent cases, a trip to the emergency room:

- Trouble breathing or chest pain
- Severe, persistent nausea or vomiting that prevents drinking fluids
- High fever or shaking chills
- New weakness, numbness, or difficulty speaking
- Bleeding, redness, or swelling at the surgical site that worsens

Practical Guidance: How to Prepare and What to Ask

- Share your full medical history, including allergies or prior anesthesia reactions.
- Mention if you've ever had motion sickness, as this increases your risk of nausea.
- Follow instructions about eating and drinking before surgery.

What to Ask Your Anesthesiologist

- "What common side effects should I expect after my procedure?"
- "Can I get medicine to prevent nausea?"
- "How will you keep me safe if I have heart or lung issues?"
- "What warning signs should I look out for after I go home?"

A Quick Checklist for Discharge

1. Mild sore throat? Normal.
2. Nausea that improves with medicine or light foods? Normal.
3. Shivering that stops within an hour? Normal.
4. Trouble breathing, chest pain, severe vomiting, or fever? Call immediately.

The Reassuring Bottom Line

Every medical treatment carries some risk, but when it comes to anesthesia, the risks are very small compared to the benefits of modern surgery. Most side effects are temporary annoyances; uncomfortable but not dangerous. Rare complications are exactly that: rare.

By knowing what's expected, asking questions, and staying alert to warning signs, you become an empowered partner in your own safety. Remember, you are not navigating this alone; your doctors, nurses, and anesthesiologist are with you every step of the way.

Knowledge doesn't just ease fear; it builds confidence. And with confidence, recovery feels less like uncertainty and more like a journey back to strength.

Part V: Special Situations

Chapter 13: Anesthesia in Children

Picture this: a mother sits by her six-year-old son in the hospital waiting room. He clutches his stuffed toy tightly and asks, *"Will it hurt? Will I wake up?"* The mother smiles to reassure him, but inside her heart races with worry.

This is one of the most common experiences parents face before their child's surgery: fear of the unknown. Children don't just need medical care; they need comfort, simple explanations, and gentle reassurance. Parents, too, need to know that their child will be safe.

This chapter will help you understand how anesthesia is specially tailored for children, how doctors explain it in kid-friendly ways, and how parents can feel more at ease before, during, and after the procedure.

How Kids Are Prepared Differently

Children aren't just "small adults." Their bodies, emotions, and needs are unique, and anesthesiologists are trained to adapt care accordingly.

Key Differences in Preparation:

- **Gentle Explanations**: Doctors often use simple words or playful comparison; "The medicine is like a magic sleep that helps you rest while the doctors fix your body."
- **Different Medication Choices**: Kids may receive a flavored drink or nasal spray before surgery instead of an IV needle right away, reducing fear.
- **Parental Presence**: In many hospitals, parents are allowed to stay until their child drifts off to sleep, creating a sense of safety.
- **Extra Monitoring**: Children are more sensitive to changes in breathing and heart rate, so monitoring is even more detailed than with adults.

Child-Friendly Explanations: Speaking Their Language

Children process the world through stories and imagination. Here are examples of how anesthesia is often explained to kids:

- **"The Space Adventure"**: "We'll give you a special mask. When you breathe in, it's like a rocket ship taking you to dreamland. When you wake up, the adventure will be over, and your parents will be right here."
- **"The Superhero Nap"**: "This medicine gives you super-sleep so the doctors can fix you while you rest. You won't feel pain, and when you wake up, you'll be stronger."
- **"The Magic Blanket"**: "The mask is like a magic blanket for your lungs; it makes you cozy and sleepy while we help you."

These explanations reduce fear, build trust, and make the experience less intimidating for children.

Reassurance for Parents: What You Need to Know

Parents often carry heavier anxiety than their children. Here are the essentials:

- **Anesthesia for children is very safe.** Pediatric anesthesiologists undergo special training to manage kids' unique needs.
- **Most children experience only mild side effects**, like a sore throat or mild grogginess, which go away quickly.
- **You'll be guided step by step.** From pre-surgery preparation to post-surgery recovery, the medical team will explain what to expect.

Practical Guidance for Parents

- **Use Honest, Simple Language:** Tell your child, "The doctors will give you special medicine to help you nap while they fix your body. You won't feel it."

- **Avoid Scary Words:** Replace "injection" with "tiny straw" or "sleepy medicine."
- **Bring Comfort Items:** A favorite toy, blanket, or book can ease separation anxiety.
- **Stay Calm:** Children mirror your emotions; your calmness helps them feel safe.
- **Report Cold or Cough Symptoms:** If your child has a runny nose, cough, or congestion, always tell the anesthesiologist. These are the leading reasons surgeries are postponed or rescheduled. Canceling early may feel inconvenient, but it is far safer than risking breathing problems during anesthesia.

Questions You Can Ask the Anesthesiologist

- "How will you help my child feel less nervous before surgery?"
- "Can I be with my child when anesthesia starts?"
- "What are the most common side effects after anesthesia in children?"
- "How will you keep my child safe during surgery?"

Quick Parent Checklist

1. Bring your child's medical history, allergies, and medication list.
2. Pack comfort items (toy, blanket, favorite music).
3. Ask how long your child will need to fast before surgery.
4. Confirm if you can stay during anesthesia induction.
5. Know what signs to watch for after discharge (like persistent vomiting or trouble breathing).

The Reassuring Bottom Line

When it comes to children, anesthesia is approached with extra care, extra compassion, and extra safety checks. Most children wake up smoothly, often asking for a snack or their favorite toy within hours.

As a parent, it's normal to feel anxious, but remember: you are not handing your child over to strangers. You are entrusting them to a team whose entire focus is on protecting children during one of their most vulnerable moments.

Knowledge eases fear. With preparation, honest communication, and trust in your medical team, you and your child can face surgery with courage, confidence, and hope.

Chapter 14: Anesthesia in Pregnancy and Delivery

Fatima (a patient) was about to deliver her first baby. As the contractions grew stronger, she gripped her husband's hand and asked the doctor nervously: *"Will the medicine hurt my baby? Will I still be awake to see him born?"*

These are the questions almost every expectant mother asks at some point. Childbirth is one of life's most powerful moments filled with excitement, but also with fear and uncertainty. It's natural to wonder whether anesthesia is safe, how much pain relief it provides, and what it means for the baby.

This chapter will walk you through the most common forms of anesthesia during pregnancy and delivery: epidurals, spinals, and anesthesia for C-sections. You'll also learn what's safe, what to expect, and how doctors protect both mother and baby every step of the way.

Understanding the Basics: Epidurals, Spinals, and General Anesthesia

Epidural Anesthesia

• **What it is**: Medicine placed through a tiny tube (catheter) in the lower back, numbing the nerves that carry pain from the uterus.

• **What it feels like**: Pressure during placement, then relief as the medicine spreads. You remain awake and aware, able to participate in your delivery.

• **Why it's common**: Epidurals are the most popular form of pain relief for labor worldwide.

Spinal Anesthesia

• **What it is**: A single injection of numbing medicine into the lower back, often used for C-sections.

• **What it feels like**: Quick, powerful numbness from the waist down.

• **Why it's chosen**: Spinals work fast, making them ideal for planned or urgent C-sections.

General Anesthesia

• **What it is**: Medicine given through a mask or IV that makes you fully unconscious.

• **When it's used**: Rare in childbirth, reserved for emergencies where speed is critical.

Safety for Mother and Baby

One of the biggest fears mothers have is: *"Will this affect my baby?"*

Here's the reassuring truth:

• **Epidurals and spinals do not make babies sleepy.** The medicine stays around the spinal nerves, not spreading widely into the bloodstream.

• **General anesthesia crosses to the baby**, but it is only used when absolutely necessary and with close monitoring.

• **Your safety means your baby's safety.** By keeping you comfortable, stable, and calm, anesthesia helps labor and delivery proceed more smoothly.

Myths vs. Facts

• **Myth: "Epidurals always slow down labor."**

Fact: While they may slightly extend the pushing phase, epidurals do not increase the chance of needing a C-section.

- **Myth: "You can become paralyzed from a spinal or epidural."**

Fact: This is an extremely rare complication. Modern techniques and trained anesthesiologists make serious nerve injury nearly unheard of.

- **Myth: "Pain relief means you won't feel or remember the birth."**

Fact: With epidurals and spinals, you are awake, aware, and able to experience your child's first moments, just without the overwhelming pain.

- **Myth: "You won't feel anything at all, not even when to push."**

Fact: Modern epidurals reduce pain but don't block all sensation. Most women still feel pressure and know when to push, which is important for a safe delivery.

- **Myth: "Epidurals are bad for the baby."**

Fact: Epidurals are generally very safe for both mother and baby. The medication is localized and used in low doses, with minimal transfer to the baby.

- **Myth: "Everyone gets a spinal headache from an epidural."**

Fact: Spinal headaches are very rare, occurring in less than 1% of cases. They typically happen only if the dura (a protective membrane around the spinal cord) is accidentally punctured, which is uncommon.

When spinal headaches do occur, they feel like a severe headache that worsens when sitting or standing but improves when lying down. The good news: they are treatable. Doctors may use rest, fluids, caffeine, or a procedure called a "blood patch," which provides fast and effective relief.

Practical Guidance for Expectant Mothers

Preparing for Labor and Delivery

- **Discuss options early**: Talk to your obstetrician or anesthesiologist before labor begins.
- **Share your history**: Mention back problems, bleeding disorders, or prior anesthesia experiences.

• **Stay flexible**: Sometimes labor doesn't go exactly as planned; trust your team to adjust safely.

Questions to Ask Your Anesthesiologist

- "What type of pain relief do you recommend for me?"
- "Will I be awake to see and hold my baby?"
- "What side effects are most common with an epidural or spinal?"
- "If I need a C-section, how will anesthesia be handled?"

Quick Checklist for Delivery

1. Bring a list of medications and allergies.
2. Ask about anesthesia options during your prenatal visits.
3. Let your team know about fears (e.g., needles, losing control).
4. After the procedure, expect mild side effects: itching, temporary back soreness, or mild headache.
5. Call your doctor if you develop severe headache, fever, or unusual numbness after discharge.

The Reassuring Bottom Line

Anesthesia during pregnancy and delivery is designed with one goal: keeping mother and baby safe, comfortable, and connected. Whether through an epidural for labor or a spinal for a C-section, today's techniques allow mothers to stay present for one of life's most extraordinary experiences.

It's normal to feel nervous. But remember, you are not alone. Your anesthesiologist, obstetrician, and nurses form a team whose mission is to guide you safely through delivery, so you can focus on the moment you've been waiting for: hearing your baby's first cry and holding them in your arms.

Knowledge turns fear into trust. And with trust, childbirth becomes less about worry and more about joy.

Chapter 15: Anesthesia for Seniors and High-Risk Patients

Eighty-year-old Mrs. Ahmed sat nervously with her daughter in the hospital waiting area. She needed hip replacement surgery after a painful fall. Her biggest fear wasn't the surgery itself; it was the anesthesia. "What if my heart can't handle it? What if I don't wake up?" she whispered.

These are common worries among older patients and their families. Aging brings wisdom and resilience, but it also brings new concerns about health, especially when surgery and anesthesia are involved.

This chapter will walk you through what anesthesia means for seniors and for people with conditions like heart, lung, or kidney disease. You'll learn how anesthesiologists tailor their care to keep fragile patients safe; and why, even in later years, anesthesia is often much safer than you may imagine.

How Aging Affects Anesthesia

Think of the body as a well-traveled car. It still works, but it needs more careful handling than when it first rolled off the assembly line.

- **Slower metabolism:** Medications may linger longer in the body, so anesthesiologists adjust doses carefully.
- **Reduced reserve:** The heart, lungs, and kidneys may not bounce back as quickly, so extra monitoring is used.
- **Memory and confusion risks:** Some older adults may experience short-term confusion (called *postoperative delirium*), but this is usually temporary.

Need to know: Aging does not make anesthesia unsafe;it just means doctors take extra precautions.

When Health Conditions Come Into Play

Seniors often face medical conditions that need special attention. Here's how anesthesiologists think about them:

- **Heart disease:** The heart may struggle with sudden changes. Doctors use gentle medications and continuous heart monitoring.
- **Lung disease (like COPD or asthma):** Breathing support is customized, sometimes using lighter sedation or regional anesthesia to avoid stressing the lungs.
- **Kidney disease:** Since kidneys help clear drugs, doses are carefully adjusted, and fluids are balanced.

In every case, the anesthesiologist's job is to keep vital organs steady and well-supported throughout surgery.

Myths vs. Facts

- **Myth:** "Older people shouldn't have anesthesia; it's too dangerous."

  Fact: With modern techniques, seniors routinely and safely undergo surgery. Age alone is not a barrier.
- **Myth:** "If I have heart or lung disease, anesthesia is impossible."

  Fact: Anesthesiologists are trained to manage these conditions and often choose safer, tailored approaches.

How Doctors Keep Fragile Patients Safe

Anesthesiologists have a toolkit of strategies for high-risk patients:

- **Pre-surgery planning:** Reviewing medical history, current medications, and recent tests.
- **Tailored anesthesia:** Using the lightest, safest dose possible.
- **Advanced monitoring:** Keeping close track of blood pressure, oxygen, and heart rhythms.
- **Team communication:** Working closely with surgeons, nurses, and family members.

Practical Guidance for Seniors and Families

Here are some steps you can take to feel prepared:

Before Surgery

- Bring a full list of medications, including over-the-counter and herbal supplements.
- Share any history of memory changes, confusion, or past anesthesia experiences.
- Ask if you'll need to adjust medications before surgery (e.g., blood thinners or diabetes drugs).

Questions to Ask Your Anesthesiologist

- "Which type of anesthesia do you recommend for me, and why?"
- "How will you protect my heart/lungs/kidneys during surgery?"
- "What can we do to reduce the chance of confusion afterward?"
- "Will I need extra monitoring after the operation?"

Reassurance for the Journey Ahead

While it's natural to feel nervous, remember this: anesthesia today is safer than ever, even for seniors and patients with medical challenges. Anesthesiologists are like skilled pilots guiding you through a short but important journey; they study every detail of your health to make sure you land safely.

You are not alone in this process. With open communication, careful planning, and trust in your medical team, seniors and their families can approach surgery with confidence. Knowledge is the best antidote to fear, and now you know; anesthesia is not something to dread, but a bridge to healing.

Chapter 16: Anesthesia for Common Procedures

When most people think of anesthesia, they imagine major operations like heart surgery or hip replacement. But anesthesia and sedation are also used for many everyday medical procedures, things like colonoscopies, endoscopies, cataract surgery, and even imaging scans.

It's natural to wonder, *"Do I really need anesthesia for something so simple?"* The answer is that these techniques aren't just about putting people to sleep. They're about making sure you're safe, comfortable, and able to get through a procedure smoothly.

In this chapter, we'll look at how anesthesia works in these common settings, what you can expect, and how to prepare.

Sedation vs. Anesthesia: Knowing the Difference

One of the most confusing parts is understanding the difference between sedation and anesthesia:

- **Sedation:** Think of this as "turning down the volume" on your awareness. You may feel drowsy, relaxed, and sometimes forget the procedure, but you're not completely unconscious.
- **General anesthesia:** This is "switching the lights off." You are fully unconscious, with your breathing and vital signs carefully monitored and supported.

For most routine procedures, sedation, or even just local anesthesia, is all that's needed.

Colonoscopy and Endoscopy

- Typically done with *moderate sedation* or *deep sedation.*

• You'll likely drift off into a light sleep, often with no memory of the procedure.

• The anesthesiologist or nurse anesthetist monitors your breathing, heart rate, and oxygen the entire time.

• Recovery is quick; most patients go home within a few hours.

What you need to know: You will not feel pain, and it's common to have no memory of the exam.

Cataract Surgery

• Usually performed with *local anesthesia* (numbing eye drops or a small injection).

• Mild sedation is sometimes added to help you relax.

• You stay awake but comfortable; you may see lights or shadows but not feel pain.

What you need to know: It might surprise you to be awake, but the procedure is quick and painless.

Dental and Oral Surgery

• Options range from local anesthesia (numbing injection) to sedation or general anesthesia.

• Sedation is often chosen for wisdom tooth removal or for children who may be anxious.

• With sedation, you may feel drowsy but remain cooperative; with general anesthesia, you are completely asleep.

What you need to know: Your anesthetic plan will depend on the complexity of the procedure and your comfort level.

Imaging Scans (MRI, CT)

• For children, or adults who are very anxious or unable to stay still, sedation or light anesthesia may be used.

• The goal is simply to keep the body still so the pictures are clear.

What you need to know: Doses are very small and carefully tailored to the length of the scan.

Minor Procedures and Biopsies

• Many smaller procedures, like skin biopsies or mole removals, are done with local anesthesia alone.

• Sedation may be added if the procedure is uncomfortable or anxiety-provoking.

What you need to know: Local anesthesia numbs the exact area being treated; you remain fully awake.

Practical Guidance for Patients

Even though these are "smaller" procedures, preparation still matters:

Before the Procedure

• Follow fasting instructions (usually no food for 6–8 hours if sedation will be used).

• Share your full medical history, including allergies and medications.

• Mention conditions like sleep apnea, heart disease, or lung problems.

After the Procedure

• Arrange for a ride home if you've had sedation.

• Don't plan to drive, work, or make important decisions the same day.

• Expect to rest for a few hours, but most people feel normal again by the next day.

Questions to Ask Your Anesthesiologist

- "Will I be awake or asleep during this procedure?"
    - "How will you keep me comfortable and safe?"
    - "How soon can I go home afterward?"
    - "Are there any side effects I should expect?"

Whether it's a colonoscopy, cataract surgery, or even a scan, anesthesia and sedation are designed with one goal in mind: your comfort and safety. These procedures are typically low-risk, short in duration, and carried out with careful monitoring.

The idea of anesthesia might feel intimidating for a "small" procedure, but in reality, it makes the experience smoother, safer, and often easier than you expect. With preparation, good communication, and modern techniques, you can walk into these procedures confident that you'll be well cared for from start to finish.

Chapter 17: The Future of Anesthesia

When James went in for his knee replacement twenty years ago, he remembers the grogginess afterward, the nausea, and a recovery that felt like a fog.

Recently, his daughter had the same surgery, and her experience was strikingly different. She woke up clear-headed, with less nausea and smoother pain control.

This is not just a lucky coincidence. Anesthesia is advancing rapidly, and patients like James's daughter are already benefiting. From smarter monitoring to more personalized care, the future promises anesthesia that is safer, gentler, and more tailored to each individual.

In this chapter, we'll look at where anesthesia is headed, how technology and science are reshaping the experience, and why you can feel reassured that tomorrow's patients, maybe even you, will have an even smoother journey.

Smarter Eyes: Technology That Watches Over You

An anesthesiologist is always by your side, but now technology is giving them even sharper tools:

- **AI monitoring systems**: Think of these like an extra set of eyes and ears. Artificial intelligence can track patterns in your heartbeat, blood pressure, and breathing in real time, alerting doctors to the smallest changes before they become a concern.
- **Personalized dosing**: Instead of giving a "one-size-fits-all" amount of anesthesia, new systems can adjust the dose minute by minute, tailored to your weight, age, and medical history. Imagine cruise control in a car, keeping you steady, safe, and balanced.

- **Better drug delivery**: New devices make it easier to keep anesthesia at just the right level, so you wake up smoothly without lingering grogginess.

Medicines Designed With Patients in Mind

The drugs of the past did their job well but sometimes left patients feeling nauseous or confused afterward. Researchers are now creating medications that are:

- **Faster-acting** (so you go to sleep and wake up more gently).
- **Easier to clear from the body** (reducing "hangover" feelings).
- **Less likely to cause side effects** like nausea, shivering, or sore throat.

For example, newer versions of common anesthetic drugs are already shortening recovery times and lowering risks, making surgeries feel less daunting.

What This Means for Recovery

The future of anesthesia isn't just about what happens during surgery, it's about how you feel after:

- **Smoother wake-ups**: Patients are less likely to feel foggy or confused.
- **Less pain, less nausea**: Thanks to improved pain management strategies and gentler medications.
- **Faster return to normal life**: Many patients can walk, eat, and even go home sooner than ever before.

A Closing Word: A Future Full of Confidence

The story of anesthesia is one of constant improvement. From James's groggy recovery years ago to his daughter's smoother experience today, and to the even gentler care awaiting tomorrow's patients, the trajectory is clear: safer, more comfortable, more personal.

When you think about anesthesia, think of it not as something to fear, but as a field that is growing with you in mind: your safety, your comfort, your recovery. The future isn't about replacing the human touch but enhancing it with tools that make anesthesiologists even better guardians of your journey.

Fear fades when knowledge grows, and in the case of anesthesia, the knowledge is full of hope.

Ending Note

Dear Reader,

Thank you for taking the time to read this book. I truly hope that these pages have brought you clarity, comfort, and above all, the reassurance that you are not alone in your fears.

Fear of the unknown is a natural part of being human. But once we begin to understand what once seemed frightening, that fear often starts to fade. If this book has helped you feel even a little more at ease with the idea of anesthesia, then its purpose has been fulfilled.

If you found value in what you read, I kindly invite you to leave a positive review. Your words can make a difference, not only by helping others discover this book, but by offering encouragement to those still searching for peace of mind.

Thank you again for your trust. Wishing you health, calm, and confidence, both in the operating room and in life.

With gratitude,

Raúl Rodríguez Sierra

www.ingramcontent.com/pod-product-compliance
Lightning Source LLC
LaVergne TN
LVHW090427210926
848480LV00002B/726

* 9 7 9 8 2 3 2 6 5 5 5 9 4 *